A Secure Faith

A Secure Faith

Knowing God's presence, power and peace
in times of crisis and uncertainty

Barbara Taylor

Mavisbank Publishing
Mississauga, Ontario

A Secure Faith
by Barbara Taylor

www.ASecureFaith.com

Copyright © 2011 by Barbara Taylor

All rights reserved.

Published in Canada by Mavisbank Publishing

Scripture quotations are taken from the HOLY BIBLE, NEW INTERNATIONAL VERSION NIV, copyright 1973, 1978, 1984 by International Bible Society. Used by permission of Zondervan Publishing House. All rights reserved.

Library and Archives Canada Cataloguing in Publication

Taylor, Barbara, 1961-
A secure faith : knowing God's presence, power and peace in times of crisis and uncertainty / Barbara Taylor.

ISBN 978-0-9868027-0-6

1. Taylor, Barbara, 1961-. 2. Cancer--Patients--Religious life. 3. Cancer--Religious aspects--Christianity. I. Title.

BV4910.33.T39 2011 248.8'61969940092 C2011-900486-0

Printed in the United States of America

Cover photograph by Barbara Taylor
Cover artwork by Jordan Anastasi

Dedicated to the glory of God the Father,
Son and Holy Spirit, without whom this book
would not have been written.

And in memory of Margaret Murphy,
my dear sister in Christ, who was there for me in
practical ways and whose own experience with
cancer has taken her to be with our Lord in heaven.

Contents

Acknowledgements

This book would not exist but for the many people - family, friends and strangers - who have touched my life from the time I was born to the present moment. To each of you I say "Thank you!" You have enabled my faith to become what it is today.

A special "Thank You" goes to my parents Joy and Will Nurse, my mother-in-law Dorothy Taylor, my husband Patrick, and my three children Theresa, Emma and Caleb, for their love and support.

I am indebted to Terry Murphy for proofing my manuscript for Biblical accuracy, to Nancy Simpson for her insightful advice and suggestions, and to David Paradi who gave me invaluable help with all aspects of self-publishing.

Prologue

What do you do when cancer, or any other crisis, intrudes on your life? You handle it the only way you know how. My way was by faith in God through Jesus Christ.

What follows is my story of faith in the midst of uncertainty, and I share it at the prompting of my Lord and through the guidance and direction of his Spirit. The experience was mine, but the faith that sustained me came from and through him, and the words that I write are his truth, not mine. I am aware that my brush with cancer is minor compared to what others have had to face and that my journey of faith is in many ways no different from that of many Christians, but I believe that God in his wisdom has a reason and a purpose for this book, and I choose to leave the outcome to him.

This, then, is not so much the story of my experience of cancer or how it affected and changed my life, as it is about the one true, eternal God - Father, Son and Holy Spirit - whose loving, living presence in my life enabled me to walk through this "valley of the shadow of death" (Psalm 23:4) without fear and with total trust in

11

him. I pray that each person who reads this will know that same faith and trust in a loving, faithful God.

The Bible is God's word of truth and has been my guide to knowing him, his will and purpose for my life and to the faith that is the focus of my story. Therefore, as you read you will find many quotations from its pages both throughout the text and at the end of each chapter. These all appear in the New International Version (NIV) for, while I still remember many of my favourite scripture verses in the King James Version, I have come to prefer the NIV for ease of reading and understanding. This is entirely my own preference and I encourage you to read any scripture references in the version of your choice.

1

Cancer Intrudes

"Peace I leave with you; my peace I give you. I do not give to you as the world gives. Do not let your hearts be troubled and do not be afraid." (John 14:27)

✝ ✝ ✝

In September 2005, at the age of 44, I developed a sore under my tongue which would not go away. With two teenage daughters and a pre-teen son, the start of a new school year is always busy so, like most mothers, I focused on my children's needs and simply ignored that sore. As the discomfort and pain persisted and it became obvious that it was in fact getting worse, I turned to prayer and a request for God's strength and healing.

Finally, accepting that God's healing might not come without medical help, I made an appointment to see my doctor in January 2006. He had no answers for me so referred me to an ear, nose and throat specialist - the earliest available appointment being in mid-March. The specialist also had no immediate diagnosis to offer and put me on a cream for a month, after which, if there was no change, he would do a biopsy. No mention of cancer was made by either doctor as I had never smoked or drank alcohol. The cream had no effect and by now the pain and discomfort were constant - like having a cold sore at its worst. I sing with the Praise Team and Choir at my church and there were some Sundays that I would

15

come home with no desire to open my mouth for the rest of the day. In fact, there were many days when the pain was only manageable by the grace of God.

By the time the biopsy took place on May 16, I had done some research about my sore and was convinced that it was lichen planus, a disease of the mouth that, while non life threatening, had no known cause and no medical cure. A friend from church suffers from this on-going disease and her symptoms and mine seemed remarkably alike, and my research on the internet seemed to confirm this. While I did not look forward to living with the constant pain I had reached the point where I just wanted an answer so that I could get on with dealing with it.

In the meantime my mother-in-law, who was living in an apartment near us, had been in hospital in early January for heart-valve replacement surgery and was recovering nicely, but we had had to place my father-in-law in respite care during her operation and convalescence, as he had been in a wheelchair for a while and was very dependant on her. While Mom continued to grow stronger following her operation, Dad's health deteriorated and his doctor was concerned about his liver.

16

About a week after I had my biopsy, his liver began to shut down and he slowly slipped away from us. Dad died in the early hours of Saturday, May 27, 2006, at the long term care facility where he had spent the last four months of his life. Those last few days were hard for Mom as she watched the man she loved and with whom she had shared 60 years of her life become a shadow of himself. Only her faith in God her heavenly Father, and the support and presence of her family, sustained her through it all.

Dad's death and funeral overshadowed my need to discover my biopsy results so it was the specialist who eventually called me on June 2, two days after Dad's funeral. With my mind expecting to hear lichen planus, it was a moment before the word cancer penetrated and my heart cried out to God, "O Lord, no!" For a split second my world turned upside down: but only for a split second. God's peace settled around my heart (John 14:27) and I listened calmly as the doctor said they would call me back with an appointment to see a cancer specialist in Toronto, and he would probably arrange to operate.

It was Friday afternoon and I was at home alone so I just sat there in my kitchen and did what I've always

17

done when I've been tempted to be afraid or worry - I talked with God about it. Having experienced his power to deal with the sin in my life, I knew that he also had the power to heal my body.

However, I did not receive any promises of healing. What I did experience was God's assurance that he loved me, knew all about the cancer, had in fact known about it from the beginning, knew exactly what my future held and would be with me every step of the way. And I discovered, as I have done in the past, that God's grace was sufficient for me, for his strength (his power) was made perfect in my weakness (2 Corinthians 12:9). What did I need to do? Trust him, just as one of my favourite scripture verses says, "Trust in the Lord with all your heart and lean not on your own understanding; in all your ways acknowledge him, and he will make your paths straight." (Proverbs 3:5-6) King Solomon wrote that, and he was considered one of the wisest men who lived.

Deciding that my husband Patrick did not need to hear this news across a telephone line, I waited to share it with him until after the children were asleep and we were alone in bed. Patrick's Mom has, in my presence, referred to him as her rock, and as the son living closest

18

to her for 15 odd years he has had ample opportunity to be there for her. That night, and in the months ahead, Patrick would be God's rock in my life - to listen, to hold me, to support me, to walk with me in faith, to be with me, to love me.

We made a decision that night not to say anything to anyone, not even our children, until we knew when the appointment with the cancer specialist would be. With Patrick's Dad's death so recent and the father-in-law of one of his brothers himself suffering from cancer we didn't want to add to the concern of our family until we had something definite to share. It is a testimony of Patrick's own deep faith in our Lord that he never expressed any anger or fear for my future.

If I could have spared my children the knowledge of my cancer at that precise time when their lives were busy with exams and end of the school year plans, not to mention the death of a grandfather, I would have done so. But life has to be faced no matter what our age and I knew that, with God's help, our family could face this. So we told them the truth and the facts as we knew them but also made it clear that we trusted God for our future. Was I going to die? That was their biggest concern

19

because I had always been part of their world and they could not imagine my not being there. Because of the killer that cancer is, and in spite of my trust in Jesus, I could not with absolute certainty answer "No", but I could assure them that God knew the answer and that whatever happened he would be with us all.

Personally, I did not fear death, for I believe the promise of Jesus recorded in John 14:1-3 - "Do not let your hearts be troubled. Trust in God; trust also in me. In my Father's house are many rooms; if it were not so, I would have told you. I am going there to prepare a place for you. And if I go and prepare a place for you, I will come back and take you to be with me that you also may be where I am." And also in John 11:25-26 - "I am the resurrection and the life. He who believes in me will live, even though he dies; and whoever lives and believes in me will never die. Do you believe this?"

Our kids are all different and some required more reassurance than the others and we tried to give them that as often as they needed it. I made sure they knew we could talk about it any time they wanted to and I prayed that they would learn to trust God through this too.

Once we had told my parents and Patrick's Mom as well as the rest of our family, we shared my news with members of our church family as well as other close friends. What a blessing to be uplifted by the prayers and loving support of so many who care for us. Many who love the Lord distance themselves from a caring Christian community but don't realize that it is through others that God often reaches out to us in love. My church family was part of God's expression of love through the weeks leading up to my surgery and in the months of healing afterwards. They, and I, are part of one body, the body of Christ, and never was this more evident to me.

Less than two weeks after I received my biopsy results I visited the Princess Margaret Hospital in Toronto to see Dr. Patrick Gullane, the surgeon who would perform my operation. Further tests were scheduled for June 22 to ascertain whether the cancer might have spread elsewhere in my body and these came up negative. However, there was a small chance that the CAT Scan might have missed something so Dr. Gullane suggested that while he was removing the tumor from my tongue he also take a scraping from the lymph nodes in my neck to check for cancer. This would involve an incision on the

21

left side of my neck which would cause some temporary, possibly permanent, nerve damage but would provide us with an answer as to whether or not the cancer was contained in my tongue. I agreed to the additional procedure and my surgery date was set for July 7, 2006, at the Toronto General Hospital. There was a very slim possibility that a tracheotomy would have to be performed but the good news was that, unless the cancer was found to have spread, I would not have to undergo radiation or chemotherapy afterwards.

There are several things that became plain to me during the weeks leading up to my surgery that confirmed God's hand on my life. The first was the incredible peace and total trust that permeated my being and never once left me during the entire time. The second was the fact that my surgeon was known to one of our dear Christian friends for he had been her brother-in-law's surgeon and he had thought highly of him. The third was the positive, confident and yet gentle manner of Dr. Gullane and his assistants as they prepared me for what to expect. The fourth was the timing of my surgery, coming at the beginning of the summer holidays and on a Friday which would mean that Patrick would not have to take much time off work and would not have to worry about organizing the children's lives as well as being at the hospital with me.

Shortly after my surgery date was set I discovered that my eldest sister Sandy would be undergoing surgery on the same day in Barbados. I had known that she was being scheduled for a hysterectomy and have to admit was amazed that our surgery dates were the same. My Mum, who lives in Barbados and had offered to come and be with my family during my surgery, was now torn between her two daughters. The choice for me was not really difficult and I had no regrets in urging her to stay and be there for Sandy. Dr. Gullane was very positive about the outcome of my operation and if all went well then my mouth, neck and possibly shoulders, would be the only parts of me affected, whereas Sandy would be recovering from surgery that would prevent her from lifting and bending and she would need assistance for much longer than I would. Added to that, God had gifted me with a husband and three children who could take care of me, and a mother-in-law who would be there for my family also.

Other than the trips to Toronto, life proceeded as normal for me and yet it was as though I was looking at life through different eyes. Although my cancer now appeared less threatening, the uncertainty of my future and the sense of how fragile life is gave me a new awareness of each day as a gift granted me by God, and each morning I was filled with thanksgiving and a deep appreciation for the opportunity to live another day. Life, my family, the very act of worshipping God, became very precious to me. It was not that I had never appreciated my life, but rather that taking the time to really consider the blessings that were mine filled me with a thankfulness and wonder that endowed them with great beauty and worth.

While others were praying for me and my family, I daily raised my own prayers for healing and strength. I believed that God would work his perfect will in my body and my life, but I had learned in my relationship with him that he cared about my inmost thoughts and desires and so I made those desires and the dreams for my future known to him constantly. I told him that I wanted to live, to see my children grow up and be part of their continuing lives, to grow old with my husband and to continue to serve God with my voice. While I am not a professional singer, singing is, and always has been, a part of who I am - it defines me in the same way that being a daughter, wife and mother defines me - and I did not want to imagine life without this special gift of God.

So I was very specific in my prayers, even going so far as to make a list. I asked for a smooth surgery with no complications, for removal of all the cancer, for healing of my tongue and the incision in my neck with no scarring, for healing of the severed muscle, for rapid return of speech and singing ability and for patience to allow healing in all aspects and not to rush things. I prayed for wisdom and guidance for the surgeon, that the cancer would not have spread anywhere else and for peace and understanding for my children. I found myself praying more for others who were sick as well - always for healing and strength and for God's will to be done in their lives.

On the day of my surgery I left home with that same calmness and peace that had characterized the past five weeks of my life - my prayers did not stop but I had left the outcome of my surgery with God. Patrick's Mom was with our children and he drove me into Toronto and stayed with me until they wheeled me into surgery. My operation was actually delayed but so certain was I that I was held safely in God's loving arms that I was able to sleep while I waited.

The surgery was successful - the entire tumor was removed. I had stitches in the left side of my tongue and the left side of my neck, I could hardly feel anything in my mouth and the lower left side of my face, I couldn't talk clearly and was very tired, but I was thankful. Patrick stayed with me for a while after I was settled into my room and then headed home to our family. I spent most of that first day and night between sleep and wakefulness. The pain when it came was slight and I was quick to do as instructed and press the button to release the necessary medication into my IV.

I had much to be thankful for over the next few days of my hospital stay. My pain truly was minimal and the staff at the Toronto General Hospital was caring and helpful. My roommate was a woman who had also had a tumor removed from her tongue but her surgery, which had taken place a week before mine, had been more extensive, and she was still having trouble eating and swallowing and had not slept much since her surgery. I have often found that God has a way of reminding us that we are not as badly off as we think we are, and my roommate's uncomplaining presence allowed me to be thankful for the things I had not had to face and to focus on my blessings rather than on what, surprisingly, became the minor discomforts and inconveniences of my hospital stay.

Swallowing food was a slow and frustrating process, and a somewhat unpalatable one given the lack of feeling in my tongue, but it was necessary if the doctors were going to discharge me. And I would have to say that my most painful experience was being poked with a needle in my hands and arms by four different nurses, when it was discovered two days after the surgery that my IV needle had shifted and it needed to be removed and reinserted. By then I could swallow medication, which was just as well since my body was so bloated that it was literally impossible for the nurses to find a vein to get the needle in.

The day after my surgery the staff had me up and moving around, and when I had no visitors I spent my waking hours walking the halls and talking with God (not aloud) or sitting and reading Paul's letter to the Romans in the Bible. Whenever I woke at night and couldn't fall back to sleep I would deliberately focus on other people I knew and pray for their needs. It's amazing how turning your thoughts from yourself and praying for others can lessen your concern for yourself.

On the next day, Sunday, standing by myself in a large hall of the hospital overlooking University Avenue, I quietly tested my singing voice for the first time and gave thanks for a "yes" answer to another one of my prayers. The words might be a bit garbled but the beauty of the music was still there and I felt encouraged that in time I would again be singing God's praise with our Praise Team and Choir at church.

I was discharged the following day, three days after first entering the hospital, and confess that I was thankful to be going home. There is something about sleeping in your own bed and choosing your own meals that is very appealing, not to mention having your family nearby. Within a week I was able to take over most of my 'chores' at home and once the stiffness in my neck eased up I started driving again.

My first follow up appointment was set for a week after my discharge and the doctors were pleased with my progress. It was several weeks before the results from the scraping on the lymph nodes in my neck were available but when they came the news was good - I was cancer free.

My surgeon did not think that I would need speech therapy and advised me instead to stretch my tongue and move my mouth as much as possible. As far as singing went, he suggested it might be at least 6 to 8 weeks before I could expect to do so. It was only as I made a conscious effort to speak clearly that I realized that God had given me my own speech therapy in my singing training. As a teenager taking voice lessons, as well as a soloist and member of a choir, I had learned to pay particular attention to my diction so that my listeners would be able to understand the words I was singing, and thereby gain a better appreciation of the meaning of the song. Focusing on my diction in my speaking enabled me to recover my speech much sooner that I might have done otherwise, although it would be many months before I fully got rid of the hissing noise that accompanied most of my "s" sounds.

Another dear friend at church who had prayed for me every day, shared with Patrick that God had told him that I would be singing again before the summer was over. His message was confirmed early in August when our Praise Team was down to one singer and I agreed to add another voice. I have not stopped singing since. In fact, during the third week of August, our church held its annual Vacation Bible School and I helped the children learn the songs. The following month I sang my first solo since the operation.

Singing has always been, for me, the most natural way of expressing my faith and my feelings towards my Lord, and when the lyrics and the tune of a song combine in such a way that they offer praise as well as declare the truth about God I find it quite powerful. Music - whether sung or played on an instrument or resonating inside of us - is one of God's greatest gifts to mankind.

Since I have not been gifted with the ability to write music I am very thankful to the many authors and composers, both of the traditional hymns I grew up with and the more modern songs I currently enjoy, who have, by their words and music, enabled God to touch my heart and revive my soul. Of the large number of songs that I deem my favourites there are several that became very special to me during the months leading up to and following my operation, and I would like to share two of them with you here.

Faithful One

Words and Music by Brian Doerksen, Copyright © 1989 Mercy/Vineyard Publishing. All Rights Reserved. Lyrics used by Permission. www.briandoerksen.com

"Faithful One, so unchanging,

Ageless One, you're my rock of peace.

Lord of all, I depend on you,

I call out to you again and again.

I call out to you again and again.

You are my rock in times of trouble.

You lift me up when I fall down.

All through the storm your love is the anchor,

My hope is in you alone."

The following song was written over a century ago, and some of the words may sound strange to the ears, nevertheless it spoke peace to my heart when Dad died and during my crisis.

It Is Well With My Soul

Lyrics by Horatio G. Spafford (1828-1888)

Music by Philip P. Bliss (1838-1876)

"When peace, like a river, attendeth my way,
When sorrows like sea billows roll;
Whatever my lot, Thou hast taught me to say,
It is well, it is well with my soul."

Chorus: "It is well with my soul,
it is well, it is well with my soul.

Though Satan should buffet, though trials should come,
Let this blest assurance control,
That Christ has regarded my helpless estate,
And hath shed his own blood for my soul.

My sin, oh, the bliss of this glorious thought!
My sin, not in part but the whole,
Is nailed to the cross, and I bear it no more,
Praise the Lord, praise the Lord, O my soul!

And, Lord, haste the day when my faith shall be sight,
The clouds be rolled back as a scroll;
The trump shall resound, and the Lord shall descend,
Even so, it is well with my soul."

I would love to fill this book with the titles of all the songs that have blessed me in one way or another over the years - songs that declare who God is, that remind me of his blessings, that encourage me to trust him, that speak of his great love and forgiveness, that allow me to declare my faith and commitment to him. Since that is not possible I strongly urge you to search out the music of Christian songwriters and artists and discover for yourself the encouragement that God offers through music.

In the spring of 2007 when the young people at our church were leading the worship service, my second daughter, Emma, not quite 15, was asked to share her story of faith during my illness, and I realized that, although her fear had prevented her from initially recognizing the peace that God had given me, living through this experience had allowed her to acknowledge God's loving presence in her own life. This is some of what she said.

"In March of last year, my Mom made an appointment with an ear, nose and throat specialist. She'd had a canker sore on her tongue for a couple months and didn't know why it was still there. The specialist had her back, and took a biopsy in May and when the results came in, in June, she and my Dad gathered Theresa, Caleb and I in the living room. She told us the results of the test, the canker sore was actually

33

a cancer tumor and she had to have an operation. I was speechless at first; I didn't know what to say. When I think of cancer, I think of a disease that ends with death, and that was what scared me the most. The thought of my Mom dying, I'd never thought about that before and then realized how much I didn't want it to happen. To calm me down, she put on a tough exterior, telling us it would be alright, even though I knew that inside she was scared too ... As time went on, she seemed to be calmer and less worried about it, showing me that her faith in God was so strong she knew it would be alright, and she didn't have to question it ... When the day finally came, my Dad drove her to the hospital where she spent three days there after the operation, during this time we went to visit her ... I can remember sitting beside her, telling her all that had happened the previous night, that my Nana had slept over and how much fun we had, that it helped us take our minds off of what was happening. When she was able to come home, she still had to rest a lot ... Even though I was still worried about her, I was thankful that she was okay, that the cancer was gone, and I wondered why I'd ever doubted it ... For me this experience was sort of a wake-up call, to appreciate all I have in life, not to take it for granted, to realize how lucky I am. I now realize that God was there all along, watching us and helping us. Even though at first it felt like he was punishing us for something. His presence was there all along."

Four plus years after my operation, most people who look at me or talk to me would not be aware that I had a part of my tongue removed or an incision made in my neck. Yet the truth is that, physically, I am different. Portions of my tongue and mouth still have either no feeling or only a tingling sensation and I am more sensitive to salty and spicy foods. Where once I sang without thought, now swallowing (I seem to have an over-abundance of saliva) and diction require a specific effort on my part. This is not said as a complaint for I am aware that this is minor compared to what many others suffer on a daily basis, and certainly it is nothing compared to the pain of the tumor and the possibility of the cancer spreading had I not had the operation.

However, the fact remains that cancer, even such minor cancer, has had a permanent effect on my body. The important thing that I want to share is that while my experience of cancer changed me physically it did not change me spiritually. Rather, it confirmed for me that with Christ on my side I had nothing to fear. Through my experience of cancer I was made aware of the strength of my faith, the depth of my trust in God and the certainty of his presence in my life.

Cancer pointed me to God - God who is faithful, loving, unchanging and all powerful - and my experience of cancer confirmed that my faith in him was secure. I know there are many others who have that same assurance. For those who don't, I pray that God will speak to you through what follows.

* * * * * * *

Additional Scripture

I have set the Lord always before me. Because he is at my right hand, I will not be shaken. (Psalm 16:8)

If the Lord delights in a man's way, he makes his steps firm; though he stumble, he will not fall, for the Lord upholds him with his hand. (Psalm 37:23, 24)

"Do you not know? Have you not heard? The Lord is the everlasting God, the Creator of the ends of the earth. He will not grow tired or weary, and his understanding no one can fathom. He gives strength to the weary and increases the power of the weak. Even youths grow tired and weary, and young men stumble and fall; but those who hope in the Lord will renew their strength. They will soar on wings like eagles; they will run and not grow weary, they will walk and not be faint." (Isaiah 40:28-31) But now, this is what the Lord says - he who created you, O Jacob, he who formed you, O Israel: "Fear not, for I have redeemed you; I have summoned you by name; you are mine. When you pass through the waters, I will be with you; and when you pass through the rivers, they will not sweep over you. When you walk through the fire, you will not be burned; the flames will not set you ablaze." (Isaiah 43:1-2) Do not be anxious about anything, but in everything by prayer and thanksgiving, present your requests to God. And the peace of God, which transcends all understanding, will guard your hearts and your minds in Christ Jesus. (Philippians 4:6-7)

2

The Beginnings of Faith

Now faith is being sure of what we hope for and certain of what we do not see. (Hebrews 11:1)

✝ ✝ ✝

The Beginnings of Faith

My journey to Christian faith began practically from the moment of my birth. I was born in the island of Barbados in the West Indies, the youngest of three daughters, to parents whose faith was an integral part of their everyday life. Raised in the Methodist tradition of the Christian Church, I learned from an early age the Bible stories of people of faith (from Abel to Noah to Abraham to Joseph to Samuel to David to Isaiah to Daniel and through to the end of the Old Testament) and God's commands of how we should live, along with the stories of Jesus' birth, life, death and resurrection, and the men and women who followed him and recorded his teaching.

I also read stories of 19th and 20th century men and women whose lives proclaimed their faith in God - missionaries like Gladys Alyward (who spent their lives serving God by sharing the gospel and giving of themselves in countries which, at that time, were not very developed by Western standards), converts from other cultures and religions (who came to faith in Jesus Christ and chose to in turn share the gospel with their own people even when it meant rejection by those they loved),

41

a young Welsh girl named Mary Jones who walked miles barefoot to obtain her own Bible, ministers like Peter Marshall, and men and women like Cori Ten Boom who lived through the Second World War, David Wilkerson who took the gospel of Jesus to the gangs of New York City, Joni Eareckson who broke her neck in a diving accident as a teenager and chose to serve God from her wheelchair, and Brother Andrew who smuggled Bibles into Russia and other communist countries.

These were true stories of people who had lived their lives by faith in Jesus Christ and had been victorious over life's situations - although according to the world's standards they would not have been considered victorious for many were beaten or rejected, lived with very few material possessions, served for years with no visible sign of having made an impact, died for their faith or did not experience the healing they prayed for.

While weekly Sunday worship and daily family devotions were an expected part of life for me and my sisters, I also saw, in my parents' lives and the lives of others who had a living relationship with God in Christ Jesus, confirmation of the truth of what I read and was taught. Their faith was not confined to one hour in a church building each Sunday but was evident in how they lived, what they did and how they treated other people. Faith, I discovered, while primarily a spiritual response to that which I could not see or touch, was also a response to the evidence of nature, the truths recorded in the Bible and the experiences of life, both my own and those of other men and women of faith.

What then is faith? Webster's dictionary lists quite a few meanings for the word but the one that most closely reflects Christian faith is "belief and trust in and loyalty to God". Webster's furthermore describes belief as "a state or habit of mind in which trust or confidence is placed in some person or thing" and "conviction of the truth of some statement or the reality of some being or phenomenon esp. when based on examination of evidence", and gives the meaning for trust as "assured reliance on the character, ability, strength, or truth of someone or something" or "to place confidence in, rely on" and "to rely on the truthfulness or accuracy of".

Christian faith is all that and so much more. First of all let me say this. I believe that faith is God's gift to us - we did not "come up with it" and cannot take credit for it. In spite of the sin that tarnishes us, we are made in

43

God's image and he has placed faith within us to enable us to respond to him and to each other. The apostle Paul says, "For it is by grace you have been saved, through faith - and this not from yourselves, it is the gift of God - not by works, so that no one can boast." (Ephesians 2:8-9).

Secondly, faith is the simple belief that Jesus Christ, God's Son, died on a cross to save you and me from our sins, to offer us forgiveness and life that is abundant and eternal (John 3:16, 10:10b, 11:25-26; Romans 3:21-24, 5:1-2a, 6:23, 8:1-4), to restore our relationship with God the Father and to transform our lives by the indwelling power of his Holy Spirit. Faith is acknowledging our sin, seeking God's forgiveness, accepting his gift of mercy and salvation and inviting him to come in to our hearts and take control of our lives.

Furthermore, faith is the certainty that we have already received what God has promised even though it has not yet happened or we cannot see it or touch it (Hebrews 11:1). It is the conviction that God is who the Bible and creation declare him to be and the willingness to place our confidence and trust in him. It is the absolute belief that God in his power and love is able and willing to do for us all that he has promised to do, in every area of our lives, even when it may seem impossible, to the glory of his name, and it is the deliberate choice to trust him completely in all things.

Jesus Christ - God the Son, God incarnate, Immanuel, God in the form of man - came to this earth two thousand years ago in order to fulfill God's promise of salvation and to make God (Father, Son and Holy Spirit) known to us. During his three years of ministry prior to his death and resurrection, Jesus not only taught people how God wanted them to live and how they could enter into a relationship with him, but he also healed people and performed many other miracles. And he always linked healing and miracles to faith: 'Just then a woman who had been subject to bleeding for twelve years came up behind him and touched the edge of his cloak. She said to herself, "If I only touch his cloak, I will be healed." Jesus turned and saw her. "Take heart, daughter," he said, "your faith has healed you." And the woman was healed from that moment.' (Matthew 9:20-22) (See also Matthew 8:23-26, 9:2-7, 9:27-30, 14:25-31, 15:22-28; Mark 10:46-52; Luke 7:36-50, 17:11-19).

45

Jesus told his followers that nothing was impossible for those who had faith and that even faith as tiny as a mustard seed (one of the smallest of seeds) could move trees or even mountains (Luke 17:6; Matthew 17:20). One particular story of faith stands out for me. Jesus was approached by a Roman centurion with a request to heal his servant and Jesus agreed to go with him. The centurion, however, declined the offer to come stating that as a person of authority all that was necessary was for Jesus to speak the word and his servant would be healed. Jesus' response was this: "I tell you the truth, I have not found anyone in Israel with such great faith ... Go! It will be done just as you believed it would." (Matthew 8:10-13)

What was the centurion's "great faith"? He believed that Jesus was able to heal his servant and he trusted him to do it, even from a distance. You see, his faith was not in the proof of the healing, but in the authority of Jesus - he did not need to see the result to believe that Jesus could and would heal his servant.

Abraham was another man of such faith and the apostle Paul reminds us of this in Romans 4:18-21: "Against all hope, Abraham in hope believed and so became the father of many nations, just as it had been said to him, 'So shall your offspring be.' Without weakening in his faith, he faced the fact that his body was as good as dead - since he was about a hundred years old - and that Sarah's womb was also dead. Yet he did not waver through unbelief regarding the promise of God, but was strengthened in his faith and gave glory to God, being fully persuaded that God had power to do what he had promised." What a statement of faith! If you read Hebrews chapter 11 you will find many brief but amazing stories of Old Testament men and women, including Abraham, who believed and trusted God.

So please take note of this - the results of faith are not dependant on how much you or I believe or how strong our faith is, but on who we place our faith in. You see, Abraham's wife Sarah did not become pregnant because he believed she would but because God said she would. And Jesus did not heal people and perform miracles simply because they had faith in him but because he had the power to do so. Nor did he die on the cross and rise from the grave because I, or anyone else, believed he would - God did that, by his choice and his power.

47

Faith, however, makes God's gift of salvation real for me and you: it allows his power to work freely in our lives and the lives of others. So, let me repeat this. Faith on its own cannot save me or change me or heal me, for while faith is necessary for God to work in my life, in your life, it is important that we understand that is it God who has the power to save and to heal, not our faith. When we can grasp that truth then we can truly put our faith into practice by trusting God to do what he has promised.

Throughout our lives, without our really being conscious of it, we constantly place our trust, our confidence, in various people such as our parents, our spouse/partner, our friends, our doctor or surgeon, as well as in things like airplanes, cars, education and medicine. Sometimes that trust is misplaced and we face disappointment or pain, but sometimes the object of our faith turns out to be deserving of our trust. For example: when I was a child, without consciously thinking it through, I believed that my parents loved me and would only do what was good for me, therefore I trusted them. So when I was ill and they took me to the doctor and the doctor prescribed medicine and my parents said the medicine would make me better, I took the medicine because I believed and trusted them. Well, putting our trust in God is similar but much more important because God will never let us down.

Over my childhood years, and into my adult years, I watched my parents trust God in the small things as well as the big things of life, whether searching for a lost item, hoping for good weather for the annual Church Fair, providing for the needs of their family, or needing strength and healing during illness. When I was eleven I made the decision to turn from my sin and follow Jesus by seeking God's forgiveness and accepting his gift of salvation. I chose to acknowledge Christ as my Lord and Master, entering into a personal relationship with God, my heavenly Father, through faith in Jesus his Son and in the power of his Holy Spirit.

In the years that followed my faith grew and deepened as I grew closer to God - my heavenly Father, my Lord and Saviour, my friend, my comforter, my source of strength and power. My relationship with God was the key to a stronger faith - the more I got to know him, talked to him and listened to his voice, the more I believed in and trusted him. Remember what I said

49

before though: the results of faith are not dependant on us but on the one in whom we put our faith. Things do not happen because I have faith - because I believe they will happen - but because the God in whom I place my faith is able and willing to make them happen.

Prayer, Bible study (both personal and in groups), listening to ministers and other speakers, fellowshipping with Christians from my own and other denominations and actively seeking God's will and guidance in my life deepened my relationship and strengthened my faith. The experiences of living - some of them amazing, some of them challenging, some of them downright awful - also had a part in shaping and strengthening my faith, especially as I allowed God to have control of the situations of life and my responses to them, and as I learned to trust him in every aspect of my life whether it was learning at school, passing exams, overcoming my shyness and anger and fear of dogs, safety while driving on the roads, what career I should pursue or who my life partner (if anyone) would be. The more I trusted God, the more willing I was to follow his leading in my life, the less fearful I became of 'what might happen' and the less worried I was about what my future might hold.

Early in my Christian journey I heard this expression and, while I don't remember who said it, it has stayed with me over the years - "You have to let go, and let God." Faith, believing in Jesus Christ, means letting go and trusting him with your whole life. Remember that verse I quoted in the previous chapter? "Trust in the Lord with all your heart and lean not on your own understanding; in all your ways acknowledge him, and he will make your paths straight." (Proverbs 3:5-6) Life doesn't often make sense, neither sometimes does the direction God leads us in, but I've learned that usually it is not my job to understand just to trust.

The year I turned 20, my family underwent a triple test of faith when my mother (a diverticulitis attack), sister Kathy (cancer) and grandmother (a broken hip) took ill within months of each other, all three requiring operations and months of recovery, and I truly learned what it meant to depend on and trust God when there was absolutely nothing I could do. My parents' response - complete trust in God while at the same time pursuing whatever medical avenues were available - to this multiple crisis encouraged me to keep holding on to God.

That summer I toured the United States with a Christian group, the Continental Singers, and it seemed so appropriate to me that the theme of the tour should be "Trust in the Lord". As I honoured God and shared the gospel of Jesus through his gift of music, I learned to entrust my family to God and trust that his will would be done in their lives. As he did with me, God worked miracles in all of their lives, although the process was long and slow.

Since then I have followed God's leading to become a lay preacher in the Methodist Church and have continued to sing his praises, I have 'fallen in love' with the man he chose for me, got married, left my homeland and family to live in Canada and become a parent. Along the way I have had to adapt to new and different people, ways of doing things and experiences. I have had reason to rejoice and to mourn, I have cried for others and for myself, I have hurt physically and emotionally, I have doubted my purpose as a parent, I have been angry, frustrated and disappointed as well as happy, encouraged and confident.

And through it all God has walked with me, and sometimes carried me, even when I chose to ignore him or questioned the paths he had led me on. Every choice I made as a woman, wife, mother and child of God, I have tried to make in accordance with his will, and in every crisis I have faced in the same capacities I have learned to turn to God for guidance and strength, trusting him with the outcome.

So then, everything I learned and experienced on my journey of faith finally led me to that day in early June 2006 when no questions were necessary and no anger or fear existed, only peace and trust in a faithful, loving, all knowing, all powerful God.

The words of the following song are very simple but, for me, they capture in a nutshell the essence of my faith.

Be Still and Know

(based on Psalm 46:10 - Composer Unknown)

Be still and know that I am God.
Be still and know that I am God.
Be still and know that I am God.

I am the Lord that healeth thee.
I am the Lord that healeth thee.
I am the Lord that healeth thee.

In Thee, O Lord, I put my trust.

In Thee, O Lord, I put my trust.

In Thee, O Lord, I put my trust.

* * * * * * *

Additional Scripture

Praise the Lord, O my soul; all my inmost being, praise his holy name. Praise the Lord, O my soul, and forget not all his benefits - who forgives all your sins and heals all your diseases, who redeems your life from the pit and crowns you with love and compassion, who satisfies your desires with good things so that your youth is renewed like the eagle's. (Psalm 103:1-5)

What does the Scripture say? "Abraham believed God, and it was credited to him as righteousness." Now when a man works, his wages are not credited to him as a gift, but as an obligation. However, to the man who does not work but trusts God who justifies the wicked, his faith is credited as righteousness. (Romans 4:3-5)

Remember your leaders, who spoke the word of God to you. Consider the outcome of their way of life and imitate their faith. (Hebrews 13:7)

3

Faith That is Secure

"But blessed is the man who trusts in the Lord, whose confidence is in him. He will be like a tree planted by the water that sends out its roots by the stream. It does not fear when heat comes; its leaves are always green. It has no worries in a year of drought and never fails to bear fruit." (Jeremiah 17:7-8)

✝ ✝ ✝

I have titled this book "A Secure Faith" because that is what faith in God through Jesus Christ has become for me - secure, established, fixed, rooted, grounded and unshakable. This is the faith that for years has enabled me not to worry (Matthew 6:25-34) and that brought peace and calm when life seemed most uncertain. Just like the prophet Jeremiah said in the quote at the beginning of this chapter, when we have faith (belief/trust/confidence) in God then we can stand strong and tall and fearless in the midst of whatever drought or storm life blows our way. Take a look also at what the Psalmist says in Psalm 1:1-3.

In the early days of my Christian journey, during my teen years, when my faith was young and more uncertain, I asked a lot of 'why' questions of God. Initially many were focused on myself. Why wasn't I pretty? Why did I have to be so shy, especially around boys? Why wasn't I smarter, more athletic? Then came the heavier questions: Why should I believe what the Bible says if, according to scholars, it was written by many different authors? Why do you allow suffering?

57

Why don't you heal everyone who has faith in you? Why do you spare some lives and not others?

God's answers were not the ones I'd expected or wanted. In fact, his answers often were not, by human standards, answers at all. His answers to me were more about acceptance - acceptance of who I was and who he is. First, I was his beloved daughter, loved by him just as I was and beautiful in his sight, redeemed by him through Christ's death, and that was the most important thing I needed to know about myself. And second, he is big enough for both of us so I had to let God be God, and that meant accepting that I would not always understand the whys of life, but not knowing was okay. As God declared through the prophet Isaiah, "For my thoughts are not your thoughts, neither are your ways my ways ... As the heavens are higher than the earth, so are my ways higher than your ways and my thoughts than your thoughts." (Isaiah 55:8-9)

I believe that God could have healed me without medical assistance. Why didn't he? I don't know, and I don't need an answer. I also know that in the course of nine months the tumor in my tongue could have grown more than it did causing more extensive surgery and allowing cancer cells to spread to other parts of my body. Why didn't it? Again, I don't know and I don't need an answer.

I learned a long time ago that this life we live and the world we live in are not perfect; they have been tainted by sin. Evil exists and with it pain and suffering. Being a Christian, a child of God, does not exempt me from life's problems but God's presence and power enable me to overcome them by faith. Faith, God's gift to you and me, that enables us to hope beyond what is seen or obvious, that focuses on Jesus not ourselves or what is happening around us or to us, that holds on to God's promises and that chooses to walk with him and in his way.

You may have heard the expression "blind faith" used with regards to Christian faith and, taken at face value, Hebrews 11:1 ("Now faith is being sure of what we hope for and certain of what we do not see.") may imply that. However, while faith is God's gift to us, I believe that faith in God is also dependent on what we know about him and what kind of relationship we have with him. I have come to know God as powerful, righteous, holy, faithful, loving, merciful, forgiving, all knowing and unchanging. I have called him Creator, Lord and Master, King of kings, Saviour and Redeemer, Sanctifier and Comforter, Father, Brother and Friend.

I have stood in his sanctuary and raised my voice in praise and known that he was pleased with my worship. I have bowed my head in silent confession for my foolish mistakes and sin and sensed his forgiveness. I have poured out my heart when I have been hurt by others or been disappointed with life and experienced his loving presence. I have come to him in anger at myself, at the people around me, at the injustices of life or at the evil of the world at large and he has borne the brunt of my ranting and raving and still loved me. I have surrendered my desire for a husband and children to him and been blessed with both when his timing was right. I have prayed for the needs of others and been uncertain of the outcome and yet assured of his great love for them. I have spoken to him out of my worry when my husband or children are late returning home and heard his voice inside me assuring me that they are in his care. I have sought his direction and discovered his leading, although not always right away or in the way I expected it.

This is the God in whom I have placed my faith - my belief and trust. And this is the God who continues to walk before me, beside me, behind me, above me and within me. This is the God who surrounds me, upholds me and fills me. This is the God without whom I would not want to face a single day of life.

In the chapters that follow I want to share with you some of what I have come to know about my God through years of prayer, Bible study, reading books by Christian authors, listening to Christian speakers, seeking God's will, and experiencing God's presence in my life and the lives of others. This is not a comprehensive portrayal of God by any means but rather a sharing of those characteristics which most specifically allowed me to experience his peace in the midst of my particular crisis.

What I share with you about God is not simply head-knowledge, it is heart-knowledge because I know it deep down in my soul, because God's Spirit lives within me and because I have come to know God, not only as my Lord and Saviour, but as my loving Father and closest friend. And while it is true that I was fortunate to have the example of loving parents to encourage me in my

61

acceptance of God in that same role, my relationship with him has gone beyond that which I share with my parents or closest friends for there are thoughts and feelings and experiences of mine that only God has been privy to.

Now before you get the impression that I think I have 'arrived' in my Christian life or relationship with God, let me state right here that I am not perfect; I have not yet become all God wants me to be; I still struggle to recognize and obey God's will; I have not yet reached the finish line in the race of life or obtained the prize, to borrow an analogy from the Apostle Paul (Philippians 3:12-14). I am still a work in progress and, thankfully, God is not finished with me yet.

What you will read is not new. It can be found in the pages of the Bible and God has revealed it to many others through their own study of scripture and life experiences. Some of the words or expressions I use may seem familiar and that is probably because others have written or said them before and they have unconsciously become part of my vocabulary. These authors and speakers from my past include Evelyn Christensen, Stuart Briscoe, Jill Briscoe, Stephen Olford, Billy Graham, Josh McDowell, Dr. William Barclay, Norman Vincent Peale,

Marjorie Holmes, Catherine Marshall, Merlin R Carrothers, the many British and West Indian Methodist ministers and Barbadian lay preachers who filled the pulpit of my Barbados church, and numerous others that I cannot begin to name.

As a lay preacher I learned that all the words God gives us to speak are not always meant for all our listeners. So I offer the following words and trust that God will fulfill his purpose through them as he promised the prophet in Isaiah 55:10-11: "As the rain and the snow come down from heaven, and do not return to it without watering the earth and making it bud and flourish, so that it yields seed for the sower and bread for the eater, so is my word that goes out from my mouth: it will not return to me empty, but will accomplish what I desire and achieve the purpose for which I sent it."

* * * * * * *

Additional Scripture

You will keep in perfect peace him whose mind is steadfast, because he trusts in you. Trust in the Lord forever, for the Lord, the Lord, is the Rock eternal.

(Isaiah 26:3-4)

During the fourth watch of the night Jesus went out to them, walking on the lake. When the disciples saw him walking on the lake, they were terrified ... "Lord, if it's you," Peter replied, "tell me to come to you on the water." "Come," he said. Then Peter got down out of the boat, walked on the water and came toward Jesus. But when he saw the wind, he was afraid and, beginning to sink, cried out, "Lord, save me!" Immediately Jesus reached out his hand and caught him. "You of little faith," he said, "why did you doubt?" (Matthew 14:25-31)

May the God of hope fill you with all joy and peace as you trust in him, so that you may overflow with hope by the power of the Holy Spirit. (Romans 15:13)

So we say with confidence, "The Lord is my helper; I will not be afraid. What can man do to me?" (Hebrews 13:6)

4

God Knows Us
Past, Present and Future

For you created my inmost being; you knit me together in my mother's womb. I praise you because I am fearfully and wonderfully made; your works are wonderful, I know that full well. My frame was not hidden from you when I was made in the secret place. When I was woven together in the depths of the earth, your eyes saw my unformed body. All the days ordained for me were written in your book before one of them came to be.

(Psalm 139:13-16)

✝ ✝ ✝

66

There are basically two schools of thought with regards to how our world, planets and universe came into existence - the big bang followed by evolution, and creation. I am not a scientist and I have no scientific proof to support my belief, but I am a believer in creation as stated in Genesis, the first book of the Bible. In the words of the writer of the New Testament book of Hebrews, "By faith we understand that the universe was formed at God's command." (Hebrews 11:3)

Initially I accepted the story of creation because it was the belief with which I was raised. However, as I thought about it, I discovered that it made more sense to me to believe that an infinitely powerful God made everything that exists specifically according to his design than to accept that our world and the creatures that populate it just 'happened'. We are different from the animals because God made us that way, just as the birds and fish and reptiles are different even if they may share some things in common.

In Isaiah 40:25-26 God refers to himself as creator of all things: "To whom will you compare me?

67

Or who is my equal? says the Holy One. Lift your eyes and look to the heavens: who created all these? He who brings out the starry host one by one, and calls them each by name. Because of his great power and mighty strength, not one of them is missing." Also in the book of Job (chapters 38-41) he speaks at great length of his creative powers, challenging Job with the words, "Where were you when I laid the earth's foundation?" (Job 38:4a) And the Psalmist proclaims, "The heavens declare the glory of God; the skies proclaim the work of his hands." (Psalm 19:1)

It is true. The beauty of the world around us, the intricacy and inter-dependence of all created things, point to a master craftsman who deliberately created a world that would support life. Have you ever gazed in wonder into the vastness of the night sky, whether twinkling with untold stars or bright with the light of the full moon? I have. I have stood on the cliffs of the north-east coast of Barbados and felt humbled by the great expanse and terrible power of the ocean stretching out in front of me, the waves pounding on the rocks below and spray misting my face. I have held in my hands many perfectly formed as well as wave-damaged shells of all shapes and sizes (as small as a grain of sand to the size of a child's fist) and marveled at their intricate and infinitely different designs. I have swum among the reefs off Barbados and been amazed at the variety of sea creatures (fish of all colours, shapes and sizes, coral, sea urchins, sea fans, stingrays, turtles) that exist along the coast of one tiny island.

Having grown up on an island it was not until I travelled across the United States with the Continental Singers that I experienced the truly wonderful diversity of God's creation. From the pounding surf of the Pacific coastline with its palm trees and beaches, to the arid, wind and water carved red-rock desert landscapes of some of the southern states, to the lush floodplains of the Mississippi River, to the wide open plains where the land seemed to stretch forever, to the majesty of the Rocky Mountains, to the massive redwood forests of California, God's creative power was evident wherever I looked.

Furthermore, I have gazed at vultures and hawks soaring on the air currents, seen an osprey swoop down and easily pluck a fish out of the water while human fishermen sat around with empty lines, watched butterflies and bees flit from flower to flower gaining nourishment and spreading pollen, peeked at a mother

69

robin feeding her babies in their nest. I have admired the determination of salmon as they swam upriver against the rapids to lay their eggs in the same place they were spawned, run my hand through the incredible softness of a dog's fur, and watched in amazement as my son's albino corn snake shed her tight old skin revealing the vibrant colours of the smooth new skin beneath.

I have planted seeds and bulbs and seedlings and watched as they grew and produced their "fruit". I have taken photographs of any number of flowers (wildflowers, tropical flowers, cacti, perennials, annuals) of many different colours, hues, sizes and form and been surprised at the beauty that can be found in even the tiniest and most insignificant ones. I have been to the zoo and marveled at the diversity of creatures that exist (elephants, cheetahs, camels, llamas, kangaroos, gorillas, polar bears, meerkats, komodo dragons, alligators, chameleons - to name a few) and that are so wonderfully equipped to live in their specific environments. Wow!

But the world around me is not all that amazes me, for I have held a baby, born of my own body, and been awed that God would endow me with the ability, along with my husband, to create another human being:

for that matter, not just one baby, but three, each one of them essentially the same and yet uniquely different.

You see, according to the Bible, God not only created our world but he also formed men and women from the dust of the earth and knit together our bodies - a skeleton of bones that is strong enough to enable us to stand upright yet light enough to allow us to move around easily, miles of blood vessels to keep every part of our body nourished and working, nerves and sinews and muscles and tendons, internal organs to take care of our body's needs, skin that stretches as we grow and that heals and replaces itself, and to top it all off a brain to control everything. I don't know all the details of how my body works but what little I know leads me to declare with the Psalmist, "I praise you (God) because I am fearfully and wonderfully made" (Psalm 139:14a).

And since God designed our bodies it follows that he must know how they work, from the blood pumping from our hearts through our arteries and veins to how our bones fit together to the cells that grow and change within us to the complexities of how our brain works. I highly recommend that you read the book "Fearfully and Wonderfully Made" by Dr. Paul Brand

71

and Philip Yancey (Copyright © 1980 Zondervan Publishing House).

Along with forming our bodies God also filled us with the breath of life and provided for us the perfect environment to make the oxygen we need, dispose of the carbon dioxide we exhale and produce the water and food that our bodies require to live. He placed within us minds and hearts and souls so that we could reason and feel and connect with him. He therefore knows our thoughts, our needs and our emotions. The Psalmist says: "O Lord, you have searched me and you know me. You know when I sit and when I rise; you perceive my thoughts from afar. You discern my going out and my lying down; you are familiar with all my ways. Before a word is on my tongue you know it completely, O Lord." (Psalm 139:1-4)

Added to all of this, he gave us a will with the freedom to make choices and decisions even if they went against his will for us. So I ask you, who could know us better, every aspect of our being, than the one who created us?

Not only does God know us intimately now, but God has always known us. The Psalmist says, "My frame was not hidden from you when I was made in the secret place. When I was woven together in the depths of the earth, your eyes saw my unformed body." (Psalm 139:15-16) He knew you and me when we were being formed in our mothers' wombs - from the tiniest fetus barely conceived to an almost new-born baby - when we took our first breath, when we crawled and stood and walked, or never made those milestones, when we spoke our first word, every scraped knee, every birthday celebrated, every hurt, every accomplishment, every failure, everyone who let us down, every hurdle we've overcome. Nothing escapes God in his knowledge of us. So, when cancer grew in my tongue, God knew about it, long before it had been diagnosed.

Back in the 1970s the word commonly used in Christian circles to describe this all knowing God was omniscient, defined in Webster's dictionary as "having infinite awareness, understanding, and insight", and "possessed of universal or complete knowledge". This might be hard for us to comprehend, but the truth is that God knows all there is to know about everything - you, me, our world and the universe.

And what about our future? We often feel that if we just knew what to expect or what the future held for us, we would be better prepared and would therefore cope better with life. Many of us know what we want out of life and we make plans accordingly but none of us really know what lies ahead or even if our plans will work out. God, however, does. The Psalmist declares, "All the days ordained for me were written in your book before one of them came to be." (Psalm 139:16) You really should take time to read all of Psalm 139. God knows what is going to happen in each of our lives, the good and the bad. He knows the people who will enter our lives, how the world around us will impact us, where our decisions and choices will take us and how the decisions and choices of others will affect us.

Also, God understands us completely because he has lived our life, or as someone else has said, "he has walked in our skin". When Jesus came to earth to live among the Jews two thousand years ago, he did not appear as an adult for a short period of time. Instead he was conceived inside a woman, was born in the simplicity of a cattle stall and experienced all that human life holds, from the vulnerability and dependency of childhood to the responsibilities and challenges of adulthood. He understands us because he has seen with our eyes,

74

touched with our hands, felt with our bodies. He has experienced temptation (Matthew 4:1-11; Hebrews 4:15), criticism, rejection and betrayal, has known physical and emotional pain, and has faced hard choices (Matthew 26:38-39) and a cruel death, "...yet was without sin." (Hebrews 4:15b)

So, nothing has happened, is happening or will happen in your life and mine that God does not know about. Instead of getting hung up on trying to understand God it is more important for us to accept that God understands us, fully. And if God knows and understands us then we can be certain that he also knows what's wrong with us and knows what needs to be done to fix it. We can therefore trust him to guide us, open doors for us, take care of us and do what is best for us, even when we don't understand.

For the one who created everything that exists and who knows all there is to know, nothing is too difficult to accomplish, nothing is impossible.

* * * * * * *

Additional Scripture

From heaven the Lord looks down and sees all mankind;
from his dwelling place he watches all who live on earth -
he who forms the hearts of all, who considers everything
they do. (Psalm 33:13-15)

The eyes of the Lord are everywhere, keeping watch on
the wicked and the good. (Proverbs 15:3)

Nothing in all creation is hidden from God's sight.
Everything is uncovered and laid bare before the eyes of
him to whom we must give account. (Hebrews 4:13)

5

God Loves Us
Always Has, Always Will

For God so loved the world that he gave his one and only
Son, that whoever believes in him shall not perish but
have eternal life. (John 3:16)

For I am convinced that neither death nor life, neither
angels nor demons, neither the present nor the future, nor
any powers, neither height nor depth, nor anything else in
all creation, will be able to separate us from the love of
God that is in Christ Jesus our Lord. (Romans 8:38-39)

✝ ✝ ✝

One of the greatest and most important truths of Christianity is that God loves the people he created. And God's love for you and me is such that he desires to have a personal, loving and never-ending relationship with each one of us.

As a child I learned that God loved me so much that he was willing to have his Son take my place on a cross and pay the price of death for my sins. God did not love me because I was good or deserved to be loved, in fact he loved me while I was still a sinner (Romans 5:6-8; Mark 2:17). No, God's love was not based on who I was or what I had done but on who he is. God is love, and true selfless, sacrificial, giving love comes from him and him alone.

The Psalmist found it amazing that the God who created the earth and the entire universe should care for the men and women he created. In Psalm 8:3-5 he said, "When I consider your heavens, the work of your fingers, the moon and the stars, which you have set in place, what is man that you are mindful of him, the son of man that you care for him? You made him a little lower than the heavenly beings and crowned him with glory and honour." I can't help but agree with him.

One morning I was driving home after dropping my daughter at school for an early rehearsal, and as I looked around me at the morning traffic a question formed in my heart. "Do you really love them all, Lord?" It wasn't the first time I had 'voiced' my amazement that God could love the millions of people on this planet and before I had completed the question mark in my mind his quiet answer "Yes" filled my soul. Why should God love us, his creatures? I don't have a reasonable answer, I just know that he does and I am awed and extremely grateful.

From the moment I believed in Jesus, and as I walked with God in my journey of faith, the assurance and knowledge of his love for me grew. I read about it in the Bible and experienced it in my own life and in the lives of others. I discovered that God loved me just as I was with all my physical blemishes and character faults, that there was nothing anyone could say or do that would change his love for me, that he loved me in spite of anything I had done or would do, and he would continue to love me even if I rejected him or situations in life made it hard for me to 'feel' his love.

The Apostle Paul wrote in his letter to the Christians at Rome, "Who shall separate us from the love of Christ? Shall trouble or hardship or persecution or famine or nakedness or danger or sword? No, in all these things we are more than conquerors through him who loved us. For I am convinced that neither death nor life, neither angels nor demons, neither the present nor the future, nor any powers, neither height nor depth, nor anything else in all creation, will be able to separate us from the love of God that is in Christ Jesus our Lord." (Romans 8:35-39) I came to know that personally. God knew me and yet he loved me unconditionally, totally and eternally.

In my teen years I was neither out-going nor particularly attractive and I struggled with my self-image. The knowledge of God's love for me enabled me to see myself through his eyes, as a beloved daughter with beauty and worth, character and purpose, redeemed, cleansed and made new by his Spirit. I was able to say with the Psalmist, "But I trust in your unfailing love; my heart rejoices in your salvation." (Psalm 13:5) I came to know that God's love would never fail me and I trusted in that.

81

I also discovered that God loved me more than my parents did, and although I didn't always see eye to eye with my parents, I did know that they loved me for they showed it in their care for me, their pride in my achievements, by listening to me and offering guidance and encouragement and support: without their saying it I knew that they would always be there for me. And throughout the years, even when distance separated us, they have continued to love and support me. I know God's love is deeper, stronger, than that. This is what he said as recorded in Isaiah 49:15-16: "Can a mother forget the baby at her breast and have no compassion on the child she has borne? Though she may forget, I will not forget you! See, I have engraved you on the palms of my hands; your walls are ever before me."

Sometimes it is hard to believe that God loves us because we do not feel his love, we do not feel his presence with us. But knowing that God loves us is not dependant on feeling, it is dependant on fact. How can knowing God loves us be based on fact? The Bible is full of both statements and evidence of God's love for us, his creation, his people. That to me is fact, and it is fact for me because I believe in Jesus Christ as my Saviour.

82

When we take that step of faith and follow Jesus as Lord and Master, when we choose to obey his commands because we believe in what he did for us, when we enter into a committed relationship with him, then God's word, the Bible, the Holy Scriptures, becomes true for us, and the words God speaks to us through its pages are fact.

When he walked on this earth Jesus said to his disciples, "On that day you will realize that I am in my Father, and you are in me, and I am in you. Whoever has my commands and obeys them, he is the one who loves me. He who loves me will be loved by my Father, and I too will love him and show myself to him." (John 14:20-21) Jesus also promised, "If anyone loves me, he will obey my teaching. My Father will love him, and we will come to him and make our home with him." (John 14:23)

Moreover, Jesus said: "Greater love has no one than this, that he lay down his life for his friends." (John 15:13) And that is what he did. Jesus has declared his love for you and me by dying in our place and his words assure us of God's love for us. That is what we can believe in.

The hymn writer, Charles Wesley, in the first verse of one of my very favourite hymns, "And can it be"

(Words by Charles Wesley 1707-1788, Music by Thomas Campbell 1825-1876), put it this way:

> "And can it be that I should gain
>
> An interest in the Saviour's blood?
>
> Died He for me, who caused His pain?
>
> For me, who Him to death pursued?
>
> Amazing love! How can it be
>
> That Thou, my God, shouldst die for me!"

The words of that hymn were written over two centuries ago, but when I sing them they still stir within me a sense of awe at the undeserved love that God offers and what it has meant in my life. Many more songs have been written and sung over the years that express the wonder of God's love, and I hope that the next time you have the opportunity to sing one you will allow it to touch your heart.

When, as a child, I complained about something I thought I was lacking, I was reminded by my parents and other adults in my life to count my blessings. There even was a chorus we learned to help us remember (from the song "Count Your Blessings", *words by Johnson Oatman, Jr, 1856-1922, music by Edwin Othello Excell*

1851-1921 - the verses of the song are worth reading as well). It went like this:

"Count your blessings, name them one by one,

Count your blessings, see what God has done!

Count your blessings, name them one by one,

And it will surprise you what the Lord has done."

How true it is that when we stop focusing on the 'negatives' we begin to recognize and value the 'good things' that are ours. And I believe that further evidence of God's love for us can be found in these 'good things', these blessings that he pours into our lives - blessings not to be counted by financial gain or magnitude of possessions.

In my case it was loving, caring parents who provided for my needs, set an example of faith and became my very best friends, a childhood that was safe and healthy, growing up on a tropical island with the sea practically on my doorstep, moonlit walks on the beach, people who taught me about God, a good education, family and friends who have touched my life, a singing voice that I could use to praise God and bless others, a job to support myself, opportunities for learning and recreation as well as service, a husband to share my life with, and children to nurture and care for. And yes, I am thankful for the material blessings that have come my way - they are part of God's undeserved gifts to me and I feel very fortunate that I have never truly been in want - but I know that they are not the true evidence of God's love.

If God loved me before I was born, if he loved me as a child and a teenager, if he loved me when I questioned him and spoke to him in anger and frustration, if he loved me when I refused to do his will, if he loved me when I was hurting so much that I shut him out - if he loved me in the past - why should I think that he would not love me now? My faith tells me that God will always love me, just as I am, no matter what I do or what life throws at me. Nothing will separate me from his love.

According to the writer of 1 John, "God is love. Whoever lives in love lives in God, and God in him ... There is no fear in love. But perfect love drives out fear, because fear has to do with punishment. The one who fears is not made perfect in love." (1 John 4:16b, 18) So the knowledge that God loves me drives out the fear -

both fear of a future without God as well as fear for my future.

Therefore when cancer tempted me to fear for my future the knowledge of God's love for me banished that fear as I trusted that God's love would only allow what was best for me. You see, even before cancer touched me God's love had already driven out fear - the fear of walking along a dark secluded pathway at night, the fear that comes from worry when a loved one is late coming home at night, the fear of losing a beloved parent who has suffered a stroke, the fear of your spouse (the family's breadwinner) losing his job. However, it goes beyond knowing that God loves me - it is the certainty that as strong as my love for my husband and children and parents is, God's love for them is far greater than mine could ever be. It is the knowledge that God cares more deeply for my family than I ever could that allows me to let go of them each day and trust their lives to him.

When I get up each morning I have no certainty that the day will proceed as I expect it to. So I commit my day and each member of my family into God's loving care and I trust him to protect us, direct us and enable us to live our lives in accordance with his will and purpose, so that we may please and serve him. I can do this because I know that God loves each one of us - he always has and he always will.

* * * * * * *

Additional Scripture

Know therefore that the Lord your God is God; he is the faithful God, keeping his covenant of love to a thousand generations of those who love him and keep his commands. (Deuteronomy 7:9)

We wait in hope for the Lord; he is our help and our shield. In him our hearts rejoice, for we trust in his holy name. May your unfailing love rest upon us, O Lord, even as we put our hope in you. (Psalm 33:20-22)

For the Lord is good and his love endures forever; his faithfulness continues through all generations. (Psalm 100:5)

Yet this I call to mind and therefore I have hope: Because of the Lord's great love we are not consumed, for his compassions never fail. They are new every morning; great is your faithfulness. (Lamentations 2:21-23)

I pray that out of his glorious riches he may strengthen you with power through his Spirit in your inner being, so

that Christ may dwell in your hearts through faith. And I
pray that you, being rooted and established in love, may
have power, together with all the saints, to grasp how
wide and long and high and deep is the love of Christ,
and to know this love that surpasses knowledge - that you
may be filled to the measure of all the fullness of God.
(Ephesians 3:16-19)
This is how God showed his love among us: He sent his
one and only Son into the world that we might live
through him. This is love: not that we loved God, but that
he loved us and sent his son as an atoning sacrifice for
our sins. (1 John 4:9-10)

6

God is Always in Control
No Matter What Happens

*Jesus said, "I have told you these things, so that in me
you may have peace. In this world you will have trouble.
But take heart! I have overcome the world."*

(John 16:33)

† † †

As you consider everything that is happening in the world around us you may disagree with the title of this chapter. However, this is what I believe - the Bible declares it and my faith confirms it - God is all powerful and God never changes, therefore God is always in control.

God's power is evident in his act of creation - in calling the universe into being by speaking a word, in forming our world from nothing and in making man and woman from the dust of the earth and breathing life into them (Genesis 1 and 2). Down through the history of the Old Testament his power can be seen in the flood that he brought on the earth in the days of Noah (Genesis 6 to 9), in the granting of a child to Sarah, Abraham's wife, in her old age (Genesis 18:1-15, 21:1-7), in the preservation of Joseph through a life of constant betrayal by others (Genesis 37 to 41), in the miracles performed through Moses in order to set the Israelites free (Exodus 7 to 12), in the parting of the waters of the Red Sea and the provision of food and water in the desert for those same Israelites (Exodus 13:17-14:31; Exodus 16 to 17), in the overcoming of armies to provide the Israelites with a new

93

home as he had promised (Joshua), in the victory of a young shepherd boy David over a giant Goliath (1 Samuel 17), in the protection of the future king David from the jealous anger of the current king of Israel Saul (1 Samuel 18 to 22), and in the rebuilding of the nation of Israel after it had been defeated and carried into exile (Ezra and Nehemiah).

When we turn to the New Testament there is continued evidence of God's power in the birth, life, death and resurrection of Jesus (Matthew, Mark, Luke and John), as well as in the changed lives of all those who followed him and boldly preached his good news (Acts).

"So what?" you'll say. "That was then and this is now." Listen: God does not change. The Creator is no less powerful now than he was when he made all things. Jesus Christ, God the Son - who turned the water into wine (John 2:1-11), stilled the wind and the waves on the Sea of Galilee (Matthew 8:23-27), multiplied the loaves and the fish (Matthew 14:14-21), healed the sick, forgave sins (Mark 2:5; Luke 7:48; Luke 23:40-43; John 8:10-11) and rose from the dead - is the same yesterday and today and forever (Hebrews 13:8). The Holy Spirit - who hovered over the waters at creation (Genesis 1:2) and

94

empowered prophets, kings and disciples down through the ages - still transforms the hearts and lives of all who come to God through faith in Jesus Christ.

At the beginning of the book of Revelation, John records this: "'I am the Alpha and the Omega," says the Lord God, "who is, and who was, and who is to come, the Almighty." ... When I saw him, I fell at his feet as though dead. Then he placed his right hand on me and said: "Do not be afraid. I am the First and the Last. I am the Living One; I was dead, and behold I am alive for ever and ever! And I hold the keys of death and Hades."' (Revelation 1:8, 17-18) Our world may have changed - with developing technology making it seem smaller, scientific discoveries stretching the boundaries of our understanding, breakthroughs in medicine allowing some of us to live longer, and developments in weaponry causing greater harm - but the God who existed before all else does not change.

King David is considered to be the author of most of the Psalms and they were written in response both to his personal relationship with God as well as to the history of God's relationship with his people Israel. This is what he had to say:

95

"You have filled my heart with greater joy than when their grain and new wine abound. I will lie down and sleep in peace, for you alone, O Lord, make me dwell in safety." (Psalm 4:7-8) "The Lord is a refuge for the oppressed, a stronghold in times of trouble. Those who know your name will trust in you, for you, Lord have never forsaken those who seek you." (Psalm 9:9-10) "In you our fathers put their trust; they trusted and you delivered them. They cried to you and were saved; in you they trusted and were not disappointed." (Psalm 22:4-5) "But the plans of the Lord stand firm forever, the purposes of his heart through all generations." (Psalm 33:11) "Lord, you have been our dwelling place throughout all generations. Before the mountains were born or you brought forth the earth and the world, from everlasting to everlasting you are God." (Psalm 90:1-2)

The Old Testament books paint a picture of God's faithfulness and his powerful presence in the lives of the people he created and chose as his own, even when they faced hardships and often chose to turn away from him and follow their own paths. Although they did not often recognize it, throughout their history God was always in control, especially when Jesus entered into their history by coming to the earth and dying on the cross. At the time of his arrest and trial, while the Jews and the Romans thought they were the ones in control, Jesus declared: "You would have no power over me if it were not given to you from above." (John 19:11)

And even when Jesus told his followers that in the world, especially as his disciples, they could expect trouble, he also assured them, "I have overcome the world." (John 16:33) Then just before he ascended into heaven he made the following statement, directive and promise: "All authority in heaven and on earth has been given to me. Therefore go and make disciples of all nations, baptizing them in the name of the Father and of the Son and of the Holy Spirit, and teaching them to obey everything I have commanded you. And surely I am with you always, to the very end of the age." (Matthew 18:18-20)

God, in Christ, has declared that he is still in control of this world that he made and I believe him, no matter how uncertain or how dark things appear to be. As James puts it, "Every good and perfect gift is from above, coming down from the Father of the heavenly lights, who does not change like shifting shadows." (James 1:17)

97

Everything I know about the God who knows me and loves me tells me that he is powerful and faithful and keeps his promises and is still in control of my life and the world around me.

And as I look back over my life I am aware of so many times when God has taken control of things that could have gone so wrong. Like the times when I have been driving and either through lack of attention or bad judgment or anger I have made a mistake that could have, but didn't, cause a very bad accident. Or when the airplane we were flying in unexpectedly dropped several feet, more than once, in an air pocket and we still arrived in one piece at our destination. And every day of life when my husband, my children and I return home safely at night I am both thankful and conscious that God is still in control.

So if God is in control, why does he allow evil to exist in our world? Why does he allow war, crime, accidents, murder, natural disasters, pain and suffering? Why does he save some and allow others to die? Why does he heal some and not others? I stopped trying to find answers to those questions a long time ago and focused on what I do know. Evil exists in our world. It came when sin came, when Eve chose to listen to Satan's tempting words instead of obeying God's command, and it has affected not just our souls and minds but our bodies and the world we live in. You see, God did not intend for us to live in a world of pain and hurt - his created world was one of beauty and harmony - but sin corrupted his world, our world.

Now I suppose God could have done away with Adam and Eve and started all over again, but the truth is, God did not create us to be puppets or robots with a computer chip that insured we would only do his will. Rather God has given us the free will to choose, and because he has done so some people will continue to choose evil. They will continue to be selfish and self-centered and greedy and rebellious as they choose to control their destinies rather than accept the grace of God and allow him to control their lives. The result is that people will continue to be hurt, our world will continue to be damaged and the same things that we use to grow and build will also be used to tear down and destroy. This, however, doesn't mean that evil is in control, only that God is allowing us the freedom to choose him or choose our own way.

Every day we make choices that affect our lives and the lives of others; choices that follow God's plan or our own desires. Some of those choices bring great good for us and for others, while other choices seem to have little effect, and still other choices bring much pain. Sometimes the choices we make are not made with the intention to harm but they do.

Often our choices are made thoughtlessly, selfishly and mindlessly, and they can have devastating consequences for other people. You've heard the stories - the drunk driver who causes death or injury to others and has to live with that guilt, the alcoholic parent and his or her abused partner and children, the drug addict mother who neglects her child. But what about the choices we make to pursue material gain at the expense of our families or others we work with? Or the choices we make to use God's gifts selfishly? Or the choices we make to ignore the needs of others?

However, the most important choice that you or I will make is the choice to accept Jesus as our Lord and Saviour and follow him. When I chose Christ, I chose to live in a covenant relationship with God, a relationship of commitment, a relationship that involved opening my heart to him, offering all that I have and all that I am to him and in his service, surrendering my life, my desires, my will to him.

And every day that I choose to live in relationship with God I not only acknowledge that he is still in control of the world he made but I allow him to control my life; and with him in control, my focus, my attitude, my priorities and my desires change, and my choices, my decisions, are no longer based on what I want but on what he wills. And when we stop fighting God's will we discover a peace, a joy, a sense of purpose, a strength, a completeness, a fulfillment, a wholeness, that will keep growing as we continue to walk in his will and in relationship with him.

Remember this, however, it is a choice that has to be made every day, sometimes every minute, if we are to make a habit of handing over control of our lives to God. It will take all of the things I've talked about before, including prayer (1 Thessalonians 5:17), studying the Bible, worship, the support and fellowship of other Christians, and deliberately seeking and obeying God's will.

101

I'd like to share with you an example of how allowing Jesus to control my life carried me in an unexpected but fulfilling direction. By the time I turned 25 I was living a full and active life, but I had come to the conclusion that I was unlikely to get married. I had talked with Jesus about it and, as I let go and surrendered this dream to him, I experienced God's peace and with it the freedom to stop 'looking'. So when love did come calling it surprised me. As a result I have never doubted that marriage to Patrick was God's perfect will for me and that our love came from God himself. Patrick is fond of calling ours an arranged marriage because we met through our parents - initially in Barbados and again several months later in Canada - but in truth we both believe that God was the one who did the arranging.

When we got married and I moved to Canada to live, many people that I met could not believe that I would choose to leave the tropical warmth of Barbados for the 'cooler' climate of Canada. Do you know something? In the twenty-two-plus years that I have made my home in this country, even in the worst snowstorm, I have never once regretted my choice or longed to return to the island to live. Oh, I confess that I thoroughly enjoy the summer months when I can wear shorts and T-shirts and go barefoot, and you won't hear me complain of the heat. Yes, Barbados still holds a special place in my heart, especially since most of my family and many of my friends still live there, and I love visiting on vacation and connecting our children with that part of their heritage. However, Canada became my home because I chose to follow God's leading and allowed him to work his will in my life.

It won't always be easy to allow God to be in control, but I can assure you of this: as a child of God the Father, precious and beloved, redeemed by Christ the Son, and filled with the Holy Spirit, God has promised you and me his presence, his power, his guidance, his unfailing love, every moment of every day in every situation of life, forever. All the promises of Scripture, beginning in the Old Testament book of Genesis right through to the New Testament book of Revelation - especially the promises of Jesus recorded in the Gospels of Matthew, Mark, Luke and John - are yours and mine to claim, for they are for everyone who, through faith in Jesus, chooses to follow him, enter into relationship with him and surrender their lives fully and completely to him.

103

God's promises are for right now, and along with his love, joy, peace, hope, mercy (Titus 3:4-7), forgiveness (Ephesians 1:7) and salvation, they include his indwelling Spirit to comfort, guide, transform and empower us (John 7:37b-39; John 14:16-17; John 16:12-14), freedom from the power of sin, guilt and fear (Psalm 27:1-3, 13-14; John 8:34-36), protection from evil (John 17:15; 2 Thessalonians 3:3), provision of our spiritual and physical needs (John 4:13-14; John 6:35) and the fulfillment of our hearts' desires when they are in tune with his will (John 14:12-14; John 15:7, 16; John 16:23-24; 1 John 3:21-22). Furthermore, God's promises are for eternity (John 5:24; John 6:40; Revelation 21:1-7).

Here are three specific promises from Jesus to hold on to right now: "Come to me, all you who are weary and burdened, and I will give you rest. Take my yoke upon you and learn from me, for I am gentle and humble in heart, and you will find rest for your souls. For my yoke is easy and my burden is light." (Matthew 11:28-30) "With man this is impossible, but with God all things are possible." (Matthew 19:26) "The thief comes only to steal and kill and destroy; I have come that they may have life, and have it to the full." (John 10:10)

So you see, on that day in June 2006 when cancer threatened to take control of my life and my future, my faith in God declared differently; and because God knew me, loved me and was still in control, I could trust him fully and completely with my present and my future.

* * * * * * *

Promises of Scripture

Trust in the Lord and do good; dwell in the land and enjoy safe pasture. Delight yourself in the Lord and he will give you the desires of your heart. Commit your way to the Lord; trust in him and he will do this: he will make your righteousness shine like the dawn, the justice of your cause like the noonday sun. (Psalm 37:3-6)

"Ask and it will be given to you; seek and you will find; knock and the door will be opened to you. For everyone who asks receives; he who seeks finds; and to him who knocks, the door will be opened." (Matthew 7:7-8)

"I am the vine; you are the branches. If a man remains in me and I in him, he will bear much fruit; apart from me you can do nothing." (John 15:5)

Now to him who is able to do immeasurably more than all we ask or imagine, according to his power that is at

105

work within us, to him be glory in the church and in Christ Jesus throughout all generations, for ever and ever! Amen. (Ephesians 3:20-21)

Therefore, since we are surrounded by such a great cloud of witnesses, let us throw off everything that hinders and the sin that so easily entangles, and let us run with perseverance the race marked out for us. Let us fix our eyes on Jesus, the author and perfecter of our faith, who for the joy set before him endured the cross, scorning its shame, and sat down at the right hand of the throne of God. Consider him who endured such opposition from sinful men, so that you will not grow weary and lose heart. (Hebrews 12:1-3)

You, dear children, are from God and have overcome them, because the one who is in you is greater than the one who is in the world. (1 John 4:4)

... for everyone born of God overcomes the world. This is the victory that has overcome the world, even our faith. Who is it that overcomes the world? Only he who believes that Jesus is the Son of God. (1 John 5:4-5)

Epilogue

Another Crisis Redeemed by Faith

Therefore, since we have a great high priest who has gone through the heavens, Jesus the Son of God, let us hold firmly to the faith we profess. For we do not have a high priest who is unable to sympathize with our weaknesses, but we have one who has been tempted in every way, just as we are - yet was without sin. Let us then approach the throne of grace with confidence, so that we may receive mercy and find grace to help us in our time of need. (Hebrews 4:14-16)

✝ ✝ ✝

Two years after my surgery, in the summer of 2008, a second crisis touched my immediate family and I once again had reason to depend on God's strength and peace. My then thirteen year old son, Caleb, woke up one Monday with a headache on the left side of his forehead that got worse during the course of the day; and by the evening he had a fever that caused him to shake uncontrollably.

A visit to the emergency department of our local hospital yielded no explanation and we were sent home with the instruction to give him pain medication and keep an eye on him. We were back in Emergency two days later and this time he was tested for Mono (infectious mononucleosis) and hooked up to an IV because he was showing signs of dehydration. As his bodily fluids were replaced there was a distinct improvement and once again we were sent home and later advised that the tests for Mono were negative.

The headaches and fever continued, and by the weekend there was evidence of swelling on the left side of his forehead. This time we took him to our family doctor who sent him for X-rays which finally showed the cause of the headaches and swelling - he had a sinus infection. Our doctor prescribed a week's dosage of antibiotics and we thought that all would now be well. The following week, the swelling was down and the headaches had decreased but he was given a second dose of antibiotics, just to be on the safe side, and sent for another X-ray.

Four weeks after the headache first started we returned to our doctor knowing that something more had to be done as the swelling had increased and the headaches and fever were once again worsening. Our doctor had expected to give Caleb a clean bill of health as the last X-ray had shown signs of less infection and he was therefore shocked at his condition.

At our suggestion and with his concurrence we took Caleb that same afternoon into Toronto to Sick Kids Hospital (i.e. The Hospital for Sick Children) where he was seen almost immediately and underwent a series of blood tests along with a CAT Scan. These revealed that the infection had spread from the sinus cavity into the skull bone and it would be necessary to operate. In order to determine the full extent of the infection an MRI was ordered and Caleb was scheduled for surgery the following morning.

One of the hardest things for a parent is to watch your child suffer and not be able to relieve that suffering. It is at those times that God's loving presence has been most appreciated. When Caleb first took sick I asked for God's strength and healing for my son, and when the pain became so bad (even though he was taking medication for the pain every four hours) that my child was reduced to tears I cried out to Jesus to surround him and uphold him and take it away.

With the initial healing came a sense of relief for all of us, but as it worsened so did our concern, and yet I still never wavered in my faith. God loved my son, just as he loved me, and he would see him and us through this. I firmly believe that my cancer experience better prepared me to trust God fully through Caleb's crisis.

Some of you who read this will be tempted to wonder why it took us so long to make the decision to go to Sick Kids. I wondered that too, briefly, when we finally took him in to Toronto and discovered the extent of his illness, then chose to discard the desire to blame myself and focused instead on what needed to done. We had come expecting an operation that would probably involve an incision and the siphoning off of the infection, and were faced instead with surgery that required the removal of part of his skull and possible cleaning out of any infection that had gotten into the brain cavity.

I admit that at that point I still did not fully grasp the severity of my son's condition, but I knew that in bringing us to Sick Kids God had placed us in competent hands and I was willing to trust Caleb to the knowledge and expertise of the doctors and nurses at Sick Kids as I also trusted him to God's loving care. This time I did not look beyond the operation to what the days ahead might bring but focused my prayers and my energy solely on the success of the surgery.

What of Caleb's feelings about all this? His life for the past month had revolved around the pain in his head and the lack of energy caused by the fever. When he felt better he had indulged in riding his ripstick or jumping on his sister's trampoline. By the time he was told they were going to operate he was heartily sick of being sick and in pain and he just wanted it to go away. Therefore, from his perspective, if an operation would take the pain and swelling and fever away, then he was all for it.

I am very proud of my son and of how he has handled every aspect of this illness. He doesn't think he was particularly brave, but he has faced without fear and a certain degree of calmness some things that would have most adults 'shaking in their boots' and very angry at life (or God). I believe that God had a hand in that as well and I am deeply thankful.

Before Caleb went into the operation I reminded him that his Dad and I, and many others, would be praying for him. His response reassured me as he asked me there and then to pray with him and I sensed no fear in him as I did so. Two years before I had faced my surgery with God's peace in my heart and there was nothing more reassuring at that point than seeing my child face his own operation with the same quiet confidence.

Caleb's operation was successful in the removal of all the obvious infection as well as the infected bone without, thankfully, any damage to his brain. His recovery was relatively quick and positive and he was soon anxious to go home. Mentally and physically he felt like himself again and he was ready to get on with enjoying his summer holidays. He was in for a bit of a shock. Because of the seriousness of the infection he was initially put on three different antibiotics, two of which he would continue to take daily (one orally and one by IV, the latter administered by a visiting nurse) for three months following the operation, and the doctor would not consider reconstructive surgery to replace the missing bone until it was certain that the infection had been completely eradicated.

However, the hardest thing for him to take was being told that, until the replacement operation occurred, he would have to wear a customized helmet 99% of the time (to cover the hole in his skull and protect his brain) and even then he could not take part in any physical activity. No ripstick, no trampoline, no bicycle, no swimming, no running, no jumping down multiple steps on the stairs. And worst of all, that horrible helmet on his head that screamed "Look at me, I'm different." He point blank refused to go back to school in September. And then he met a girl, not much younger than himself, who had no hair as a result of her cancer treatments but who was excited about, even looking forward, to going back to school. That changed his outlook. Coincidence? I believe God used that girl without her knowing it to work a change in my son. By the time school came around Caleb was comfortable enough with his helmet to talk to his class about his whole experience and would even tell his story to anyone who asked a question or made a comment about his helmet.

Now, I'm not saying that he was a model 'patient'. A growing teenage boy is a bundle of energy and my son was no different. I believe it was only by the grace of God (television, electronic games and walking to and from school also helped) that he and I made it through the following months without tearing our hair out and without any further damage to his head. To give him his due he was pretty good at following the rules although I can't be absolutely certain about when he was out of my sight. Twice he faced disappointment as the projected times for the second operation were put back, but finally the day came in mid February 2009, eight months after the first operation, when he returned to Sick Kids Hospital "to have his head fixed".

This time we were more mentally prepared - we had a better knowledge and understanding of the possible dangers inherent in the operation as well as what to

115

expect following the surgery. Also there were many more people praying for a good outcome. Once again we placed our trust in God and committed the outcome of the surgery to him, and once again God granted us his peace. Caleb came through another successful operation and we gave thanks for the skill of his surgeon and the other doctors and nurses at Sick Kids. All of the staff at Sick Kids were truly wonderful and our son was soon well on the way to recovery. Two plus years later the only evidence of his trauma is a scar that is hidden by his hair.

So tell me this: should I have asked God, "Why did you allow this to happen to my son?" Surely the more important questions should be, "How come, after four weeks, the infection didn't get into his brain?" or "What if we hadn't lived so near to a hospital like Sick Kids and he hadn't been able to get the help he needed? What might have been the outcome then?" You see God worked a miracle in my son's life with the help of some very skilled and dedicated and caring people, and I am very thankful that he is whole again, physically and mentally. However, even more precious to me was the experience of God's loving and sustaining presence through it all and the knowledge that Caleb has matured as a person through his experience.

How will you handle the crises in your life - in your own strength, or with God's grace and peace and loving presence? I know I could never have done it on my own and not become bitter and unhappy. God loves you - more than you could ever imagine. He knows all there is to know about you and he wants you to allow him to have control of your life so that you may experience his mercy, his life-changing power and all the abundance of his promises and blessings. But the choice is yours. I can promise you this however - if you let him into your heart and you commit your whole life to him and you walk in relationship with him, he will never leave you or forsake you.

Psalm 23

The Lord is my shepherd, I shall not be in want.

He makes me lie down in green pastures,

he leads me beside quiet waters, he restores my soul.

He guides me in paths of righteousness

for his name's sake.

Even though I walk through the valley

of the shadow of death,
I will fear no evil, for you are with me;
your rod and your staff, they comfort me.
You prepare a table before me
in the presence of my enemies.
You anoint my head with oil; my cup overflows.
Surely goodness and love will follow me
all the days of my life,
and I will dwell in the house of the Lord forever.